CONTENTS

1

CHECK UP ON
YOUR DOCTOR

DEADLY MISTAKES THAT DOCTORS MAKE

Source: **Paul Barach, MD, MPH,** director of strategic planning for patient safety, associate professor of anesthesiology, associate dean for patient safety and quality improvement, all at the University of Miami School of Medicine. He led the effort in Florida to create the Florida Patient Safety Corporation.

When Dr. Paul Barach was a third-year medical student, an attending physician told him to insert a central intravenous (IV) line into a 75-year-old patient suffering from emphysema. Dr. Barach had never performed the procedure before. Alone and unguided, he wound up puncturing the air sac around the lung, and the patient eventually died of related complications.

Though Dr. Barach went on to an illustrious career, he was haunted by the incident and became driven to understand how medical errors can be prevented. Today, Dr. Barach is one of the country's foremost patient-safety advocates.

We recently spoke with him about the best ways for medical consumers to protect themselves against medical errors.

What are the most common errors?

Medication errors. This includes not only oral medications but also errors involving IV drugs (given through the veins for serious conditions, such as heart attack or stroke) or subcutaneous injections (given beneath the skin, such as a diabetic's insulin shot). The Institute of Medicine estimates that 3% to 5% of all medication is administered incorrectly.

Medication errors include a number of different scenarios and can happen anywhere—in hospitals, doctors' offices and pharmacies. For example, a drug may not be given at exactly the right time, in the right dose or with the right frequency. In most instances, this type of error is minor and has no consequences.

However, IV drugs act much more quickly than oral medications, so those mistakes are frequently irreversible and the consequences are more severe. With chemotherapy, for example, dosing is a very complex process that requires different combinations and amounts of toxic drugs, so there's an even greater risk for harm.

Are certain people at increased risk for medical errors?

Older adults and psychiatric patients all are at high risk. Older adults are more likely to be on multiple medications and less likely to pay close attention when drugs are being administered. Psychiatric patients generally don't ask questions related to medications.

What can patients do to make sure their medication is being administered properly?

Get very clear and very detailed explanations from your provider, beforehand and in writing. Find out what you're going to be taking, for how long and what side effects might occur. Using a polite tone, ask your physician, *Can you please tell me what this drug is for? What are its side effects? What dose should I be on?* Research the medication(s) before you take them. Read about them in a medical reference book at your local library, surf the Internet or talk to your pharmacist. Then make sure you get what you are prescribed. If you have any doubts or questions whatsoever, be sure to speak up.

How can patients protect themselves before they undergo anesthesia?

Patients should insist on meeting their anesthesiologist ahead of time to discuss all of their concerns and to go through their complete medical history. You cannot assume that your anesthesiologist has your records or has reviewed them.

Mention if you or a family member has had trouble with anesthesia or if you have a history of hyperthermia (a rare condition in which the body is susceptible to very high fevers).

Also mention if you have any loose teeth. In rare cases, a patient's teeth are knocked out when the breathing tube is inserted down the throat. Teeth are nicked, chipped or broken in about 500 of 100,000 cases. That's about 0.5% of the time.

A good hospital will always require you to have a preoperative examination with an anesthesiologist. This is the only person who understands how to monitor your medications.

We all know that hospital patients should ask a family member or friend to be on-site to help monitor their care. What should this person be looking for?

Your guardian should know your treatment plan and your medication schedule. He/she should ask your doctor about these facts and write them down. If the doctor has put you on a low-sodium diet, for example, your guardian should ask if the food is low-sodium when it arrives. Your guardian should scrutinize any medicine before it is administered to make sure it's correct. This is especially true if, for example, the patient in the next room has a name that is similar to yours.

What's the best way to choose a care guardian?

Look for someone with common sense, inquisitiveness and assertiveness. Choose a person who will put your interests above everything else and who will be able to stand up for you should a discrepancy arise.

If a health-care provider appears incompetent, should a patient insist on having someone else take over?

That depends. If someone is causing you unusual pain or prodding or poking you too hard during an examination, you should alert the head nurse or attending physician. You even can get up and leave, if necessary.

Sometimes a caregiver can have trouble performing a procedure through no fault of his own. Even the most experienced health-care professional can take 45 minutes to get an IV line into a long-term smoker whose veins are hardened.

If you feel that you are not receiving the caregiver's undivided attention or if there is a lot of noise and confusion in your room, voice your concern.

How common is it for people to die or for serious errors to occur without the patient or family members knowing what went wrong?

No one knows for sure. If you believe that a medical error has occurred, talk to your caregiver. Ask for a full disclosure of all the facts and a copy of your medical records and charts. If necessary, you can ask to speak to the head of the department. If you still are not getting an adequate response or if you feel you are being stonewalled, contact the head of the hospital.

Documentation has greatly improved over the years, providing more accountability in case of a medical error.

■

WHEN TO SAY "NO!" TO YOUR DOCTOR

Source: **Charles B. Inlander,** a consumer advocate and health-care consultant based in Fogelsville, PA. He is author of more than 20 books on consumer health issues, including *Take This Book to the Hospital with You: A Consumer Guide to Surviving Your Hospital Stay.* St. Martin's.

It may sound strange, but saying "no" to your doctor may improve your health. Don't get me wrong. I'm not suggesting you become an obstinate, bullheaded patient just for the fun of it. Instead, saying "no" is a tactic savvy health-care consumers use to get the information they need to make an informed medical or health decision. **SAY "NO" IF...**

• *Your doctor proposes an invasive procedure without discussing alternatives.* Whether it's major surgery or a risky treatment, such as chemotherapy, your doctor should explain all your options as well as the risks and possible benefits of the proposed procedure or treatment. Several years ago, I helped an 80-year-old man whose doctor told him he "must" have his cancerous prostate gland surgically removed. I advised this man to say "no" until the doctor disclosed the risks, benefits and alternatives to the operation. When he did so, the doctor said that at his patient's age there were significant risks, the benefits would probably be minimal and that alternatives, such as injected medication, were available. The gentleman chose this alternative and is still alive today.

• *Your doctor proposes a medical test without explaining why.* Before agreeing to a medical test, you should be told why it needs to be done, what the doctor expects to find and what, if anything, can be done when the results are determined. Although many tests are important, some studies show that up to half of all medical tests are unnecessary. Some verge on downright medical malpractice. For example, I recently helped a family file a complaint with their state medical licensing board against a doctor who repeatedly ordered painful medical tests for their aunt who was terminally ill with a malignant brain tumor. When asked to stop, he insisted it was important to monitor her condition. Yet, no matter what the tests found, there were no treatments that would make her better.

• *Your doctor tries to dissuade you from getting a second opinion.* Studies show that about 20% of all diagnostic second opinions (those attempting to verify what's wrong with you) do not agree with the first opinion. The percentage is even higher for second opinions regarding treatment for a diagnosed condition. Any doctor who discourages a second opinion is not to be trusted. In fact, you may even want to get a third opinion if the doctors you've consulted disagree.

■

HEART DISEASE: WHAT WOMEN—AND THEIR DOCTORS—OFTEN OVERLOOK

Source: **Nieca Goldberg, MD,** a cardiologist and former chief of Women's Cardiac Care at Lenox Hill Hospital in New York City. She is assistant clinical professor of medicine at New York University School of Medicine, and author of *Women Are Not Small Men: Life-Saving Strategies for Preventing and Healing Heart Disease in Women* (Ballantine) and *The Women's Healthy Heart Program* (Random House). *www.totalheartcare.com.*

Most women now know that heart disease is their single greatest health risk—greater than stroke and all cancers, including breast malignancies, combined.

However, many doctors still associate heart disease with men—and overlook it in women. That's partially because a woman's symptoms of heart disease or a heart attack are different from symptoms in men—but no less dangerous.

Consider these facts...

• *A woman has a one in two lifetime risk of dying from heart disease.* (Her lifetime risk of dying from breast cancer is only one in 25.)

• *Women are twice as likely as men to die in the first few weeks following a heart attack.*

Fortunately, recent research has revealed ways to help protect women.

DELAYED ONSET...

Heart disease in women tends to become apparent about 10 years later than it does for men. The same risk factors that cause men to have heart attacks in middle age are initially masked in women by the protective effects of estrogen, the hormone that is associated with healthy cholesterol levels. After menopause, sharp declines in estrogen dramatically increase a woman's risk for heart attack.

DIFFERENT SYMPTOMS...

The "classic" heart attack symptoms, such as crushing chest pain or pain that radiates down an arm, can affect women, but are more common in men. Women have their own classic symptoms, which doctors often fail to recognize. THEY INCLUDE...

• *Unusual fatigue.*
• *Heart palpitations.*
• *Pressure or pain* in the upper abdomen.
• *Back pain* or symptoms resembling indigestion.

Angina, mild to severe chest pain caused by insufficient blood to the heart and often the initial symptom of a heart attack, occurs less often in women than in men. Women are more likely than men to suffer *angina-equivalent* symptoms—shortness of breath, tightness or tingling in the arm and/or lower chest.

Doctors who don't recognize heart attack symptoms in women may delay lifesaving treatments—and women may not go to a hospital because they don't understand the significance of the symptoms.

MISSED RISK FACTORS...

About 80% of women who die suddenly of a heart attack have modifiable risk factors, such as obesity or a history of smoking, but women are less likely to receive adequate counseling regarding preventive strategies.

IMPORTANT: Because heart disease is strongly associated with lifestyle issues, women must begin addressing key risk factors, such as weight, exercise levels, diabetes and smoking, years before menopause.

DIFFERENT LIPID PROFILES...

Elevated cholesterol levels can be associated with heart disease in men as well as in women—but elevated levels of blood fats known as triglycerides present a greater risk for women, even when their cholesterol levels are low. Women with high triglycerides also tend to have high total and low-density lipoprotein (LDL) cholesterol, and low levels of high-density lipoprotein (HDL) cholesterol.

RECOMMENDATION 1: A woman's triglycerides should be less than 150 mg/dL. Her HDL should be 50 mg/dL or higher, and her LDL should be less than 100 mg/dL. In men, triglycerides and LDL levels should be the same, and HDL should be 40 mg/dL or higher.

A recent study published in the journal *Circulation* found that nearly two-thirds of women at very high risk for heart disease had unacceptably high levels of cholesterol, but only about one-third were receiving statins or other appropriate medication, as recommended by the American Heart Association.

RECOMMENDATION 2: Every woman age 20 or older should ask her doctor for a fasting lipoprotein profile, which measures total, LDL and HDL cholesterol, along with triglycerides (a 12-hour fast ensures that triglycerides are not falsely elevated). If the first test is normal, repeat it in five years. Abnormal tests are usually repeated in six months to a year, following medicine or lifestyle changes to control cholesterol and triglyceride levels.

INSUFFICIENT TESTING...

When women undergo angiography, an imaging test that examines the blood vessels of the heart, doctors usually find that they have fewer diseased arteries than the typical male patient—yet women have a higher death rate from heart disease. This is primarily because women often have other conditions, such as hypertension, diabetes or even heart failure, that increase risk for heart attack and stroke but aren't treated as aggressively as they are in men.

IMPORTANT: Every woman should know her blood pressure...her cholesterol levels...and other heart disease risk factors. If her doctor doesn't routinely order these tests—and recommend treatment when required—she should insist on it.

A standard test for heart disease is the exercise stress test, in which a person walks on a treadmill while being monitored by an electrocardiogram (ECG), a test that measures the electrical activity of the heartbeat.

The stress test increases the work of the heart and reveals angina or other symptoms that are present only during exertion. The test can help detect coronary artery disease in men about 90% of the time—but for reasons that are not yet known, it is not as accurate in women.

In about half of cases, women with coronary artery disease who receive an ECG during a stress test will appear to have normal coronary arteries. This false-negative reading may occur if a woman doesn't achieve a high enough heart rate during the test, or if beta blocker or other medications she's taking keep her heart rate artificially low.

IMPORTANT: Women with heart disease symptoms should get a stress test that includes imaging studies, such as a nuclear exercise stress test (which involves the injection of a radioactive substance to produce images of the heart muscle) or an exercise echocardiogram (which uses ultrasound waves to view the heart). These tests provide more accurate results and are typically covered by insurance.

ASK ABOUT ASPIRIN...

Doctors routinely recommend aspirin therapy for patients with an elevated risk for heart disease.

NEW FINDING: Aspirin does not reduce the risk for heart attack in healthy women under age 65...and is more likely to cause gastrointestinal upset or bleeding problems in women than in men. In women over age 65, the heart benefits of aspirin may outweigh the risks for stomach problems.

In my opinion, women with heart disease or risk factors benefit from taking aspirin. Get your doctor's advice before starting aspirin therapy.

OVERLOOKED STRESS...

Women often must balance more life roles and responsibilities than men but may feel that they have less control at home or in the workplace. This situation can foster anxiety, anger or depression, all of which are major risk factors for heart disease, according to reliable scientific studies.

Elevated stress hormones, particularly cortisol and adrenaline, raise blood pressure and/or heart rate. Elevated cortisol levels also increase the coronary arteries' susceptibility to plaque buildup. Central adiposity, a condition associated with elevated cortisol and characterized by accumulations of abdominal fat, greatly increases heart disease risk.

Women with untreated depression and/or high levels of anxiety or stress should talk to a counselor or therapist. Social support also helps.

In a recent pilot study, women with heart disease participated in either coed exercise sessions using weight machines...or joined a women-only aerobics class. Levels of depression and anxiety were significantly decreased in the aerobics group, probably because of the social support the women got from working out with each other.

■

STRESS TESTS ARE NOT FOOLPROOF

Source: **Mehmet C. Oz, MD,** director, Cardiovascular Institute, Columbia University Medical Center, New York City. He is coauthor of *You: The Owner's Manual.* HarperCollins.

Signs of heart disease can be missed by exercise stress tests. An exercise stress test, which consists of an electrocardiogram (ECG) and blood pressure measurement while exercising on a treadmill, is commonly used to identify heart problems. However, stress tests fail to identify high risk for heart attack in 25% of patients.

SELF-DEFENSE: To increase accuracy to 90%, ask your doctor also to perform a thallium scan and echocardiogram.

■

WARNING: READ THIS BEFORE HAVING OUTPATIENT SURGERY

Source: **Charles B. Inlander,** a consumer advocate and health-care consultant based in Fogelsville, PA. He is author of more than 20 books on consumer health issues, including *Take This Book to the Hospital with You: A Consumer Guide to Surviving Your Hospital Stay.* St. Martin's.

Few things in medicine have changed more radically in the past 20 years than the places people go for surgery. More than 1,500 different surgical procedures that previously were performed only on an inpatient basis, including the removal of cataracts and colon polyps, now can be performed on outpatients who enter a facility in the morning and leave later the same day. Although outpatient surgeries are cheaper and often safer (largely because of significantly lower infection rates), a successful outcome typically depends on the type of outpatient facility you choose for your procedure.

Key points to consider...

• *Doctors' offices.* You are not paying the high overhead associated with a hospital or free-standing surgical center, so procedures performed in a doctor's office can cost up to 50% less than those in the other settings—but they come with greater risk. That's because doctors' offices are not accredited by any private or government oversight agency. In fact, under current state laws, any licensed doctor (physicians must be licensed by the state in which they practice) can perform just about any surgical procedure in his/her own office without any special approval. Because of this, insurance companies and Medicare may not pay for a procedure performed in a physician's office. Check to see if your insurer will pay for the procedure you need with the doctor you are considering. If not, ask the company for a list of doctors' offices approved for payment.

• *Free-standing surgical centers.* Often called "surgi-centers," these usually are a better choice than a doctor's office. These facilities, often independently owned by physicians or entrepreneurs, tend to be better regulated. Most states require them to be licensed, usually by the state health department. That means they are inspected and must meet certain standards for safety, infection control and other quality-related factors.

They also can be accredited by the Accreditation Association for Ambulatory Healthcare or the Joint Commission on the Accreditation of Healthcare Organizations. Although accreditation is voluntary for surgi-centers, it's smart to choose a facility that is accredited by one of these organizations.

• *Hospital-owned outpatient facility.* This usually is your best choice for outpatient surgery. Since it is a part of a hospital, it must meet the same regulatory standards and accreditation requirements as the rest of the hospital (even if it is not located at the hospital site). These standards and requirements are much more strict and comprehensive than for other settings. Unlike a doctor's office or a surgi-center, hospital-owned outpatient facilities collect important data, such as infection rates. Many hospitals now are making that information publicly available. Ask for the annual surgical and outpatient report. If it's not available, consider another facility.

■

NURSING SHORTAGE MAY LEAD TO MORE MISTAKES

Source: **Charles B. Inlander,** a consumer advocate and health-care consultant based in Fogelsville, PA. He is author of more than 20 books on consumer health issues, including *Take This Book to the Hospital with You: A Consumer Guide to Surviving Your Hospital Stay.* St. Martin's.

Not long ago, I received a letter from a man who complained that he never saw the same nurse twice during the five days he was recently hospitalized. During one of those days, the consequences were almost deadly when a nurse came into his room to give him a medicine to which he was allergic. Because he had never seen the nurse—nor was scheduled to receive any pills—he refused to take the medication. She later returned and apologized, telling him that because of the hospital's nurse shortage, she had been assigned to work a floor that was new to her and she had entered the wrong room.

The nurse shortage in the US is severe. The American College of Healthcare Executives recently found that 72% of hospital CEOs reported nurse shortages at their facilities. The effect of this shortage is felt most acutely in hospitals, assisted-living facilities and nursing homes.

A study in *The New England Journal of Medicine* found that 53% of doctors cited the nurse shortage as a leading cause of medical errors. Even so, nursing-school enrollments are not large enough to fill the gap anytime soon. **HERE'S HOW TO PROTECT YOURSELF...**

• *Ask about nurse-to-patient ratios.* In hospitals, there should be at least one registered nurse (RN) at all times for every six medical or surgical patients. In the intensive-care unit, emergency room and labor/delivery area, the ratio should be one RN for every two patients. Skilled-nursing homes should have an RN on duty at all times and at least one licensed practical nurse (LPN) for every 10 patients. Assisted-living facilities always should have at least one RN on site and an adequate number of aides to meet the medical needs that arise. Call the nurse administrator at the hospital, assisted-living facility or nursing home and ask for their ratios. If a facility exceeds the numbers listed above, consider finding an alternative.

• *Keep a log.* Because you may not see the same nurse very often, it is important for you or a family member to keep track of your care. Keep a list of the medications your doctor has ordered and the times you should receive them. When you're administered the drugs, record the times and dosage in a log. Write down the time and results when someone takes your blood pressure or temperature. Include the name of every nurse or aide who treats you and note the date, time and what he/she did. Keeping your own record lowers the chance of error.

• *When in doubt, just say no!* Refuse to take or do anything you're not sure about. This includes medicines and tests, especially if presented by someone you've never seen. Ask for your doctor's confirmation.

• *Call for help.* If a nurse is not responding to your call button and you need immediate help, pick up the phone and ask the operator to connect you to the nursing station on your floor. Someone *will* answer—say you need assistance at once.

■

BE SURE YOUR SURGEON KNOWS WHERE TO CUT

Source: **Richard Croteau, MD,** executive director for patient safety initiatives, Joint Commission International Center for Patient Safety, Oakbrook Terrace, IL.

Incision sites must now be marked by surgeons. The new US rules, established by the Joint Commission on Accreditation of Healthcare Organizations, also require the surgical team to take a "time-out" before starting surgery. This ensures that the right patient is on the table and that all doctors, nurses and other medical personnel agree on what procedure is to be performed. Mistakes, such as operating on the wrong side of a patient or performing the wrong procedure, were reported about 300 times from 1995 to 2004.

IF YOU'RE UNDERGOING SURGERY: Ask your surgeon to mark the surgical site when you are awake. Otherwise, ask a friend or family member to observe.

UNEXPECTED SOURCES OF LETHAL INFECTIONS

Source: **Charles B. Inlander,** a consumer advocate and health-care consultant based in Fogelsville, PA. He is author of more than 20 books on consumer health issues, including *Take This Book to the Hospital with You: A Consumer Guide to Surviving Your Hospital Stay.* St. Martin's.

Some people may be aware of the dangers of deadly infections acquired in hospitals. According to the Centers for Disease Control and Prevention (CDC), these infections kill approximately 100,000 patients each year, seriously harm almost 2 million additional people and add more than $5 billion to annual health-care costs. The CDC also estimates that up to half of these infections are preventable, if only hospital personnel would take infection control more seriously—primarily by washing their hands.

However, hospitals aren't the only place where unsuspecting medical consumers can acquire deadly infections. You also can get an infection at outpatient surgical and emergency centers, nursing homes, assisted-living facilities—even in your doctor's office. Not a single state routinely inspects nonhospital medical facilities for infection-control practices, nor do states require these facilities to report infections that might have been caused by treatments received there. That means it's up to you—the patient—to take steps that will lower your risk for infection. **BEST STRATEGIES...**

• *Look for clean hands.* You may have heard it before, but you cannot afford to ignore this advice. In fact, the CDC reports that staff not washing their hands is the number-one reason that infections spread. Don't let anyone—not even a doctor or a nurse—touch you unless he/she has washed his hands in your presence. If a health-care worker comes into the examining room with gloves on, ask him to remove those gloves, wash his hands and put on new gloves. It's been found that, in rare cases, personnel wear the same gloves all day long!

• *Insist on clean equipment.* For example, make sure a doctor or nurse wipes the flat surface (diaphragm) of his stethoscope with alcohol before listening to your chest. Studies show that stethoscopes can be contaminated with *Staphylococcus aureus* and other deadly bacteria that can easily spread if the equipment is not cleaned.

• *Beware of urinary catheters.* Infections caused by urinary catheters are a problem, especially in nursing homes and assisted-living facilities. The longer the catheters stay in, the greater the risk for infection. Too often catheters are inserted in patients for the convenience of the staff, simply because they do not have the time (or desire) to bring a bedpan or change a diaper. Unless there is a medical reason for a urinary catheter, insist on a bedpan or diaper. It can save your life—or that of a loved one.

• *Ask about presurgical antibiotics.* When it comes to infection, outpatient surgery is just as risky as inpatient surgery. Research now shows that many patients should be given an antibiotic within one hour of surgery. Unfortunately, busy health-care workers often forget to administer it. So when your surgery is scheduled, talk to your doctor about receiving a presurgical antibiotic. If it is recommended, ask about the antibiotic as soon as you arrive at the facility or doctor's office.

■

PROTECT YOURSELF

WHAT YOUR DOCTOR ISN'T TELLING YOU: HOW TO PREVENT CANCER

Source: **Richard S. Rivlin, MD,** professor of medicine at Weill Medical College of Cornell University and director, Anne Fisher Nutrition Center at Strang Cancer Prevention Center, both in New York City. He is also a consultant at Memorial Sloan-Kettering Cancer Center in New York City.

Cancer claims the lives of 1,500 Americans each day. But up to two-thirds of these malignancies could be prevented.

Millions of Americans have taken cancer prevention to heart and made lifestyle changes—eating a nutritious diet, maintaining a healthful weight and not smoking. Now, the latest cancer research has identified other important prevention strategies that most people don't take seriously enough.

Key mistakes…

1. *Inhaling secondhand smoke.* Each year, tobacco use causes approximately 180,000 cancer deaths. Millions of Americans have quit smoking, but most people underestimate the risk of even occasional exposure to secondhand smoke.

The Environmental Protection Agency (EPA) estimates that secondhand smoke causes approximately 3,000 cases of lung cancer in the US annually. If you live with someone who smokes, your risk of dying from lung cancer is 30% higher than if you live in a smoke-free environment.

SELF-DEFENSE: Avoid secondhand smoke by asking guests to smoke outside, for example, or staying away from groups of smokers outside office buildings. This will immediately reduce your risk for cancers of the lung, throat, bladder, kidney, pancreas and mouth.

BONUS: A recent study in the *British Medical Journal* reported that hospital admissions for heart attacks dropped by 60% in Helena, Montana, when the city adopted a smoke-free policy. As little as 30 minutes of exposure to secondhand smoke is hazardous to people with heart or lung conditions.

2. *Not getting annual skin exams.* There are about one million cases of non-melanoma skin cancer diagnosed annually in the US—plus more than 54,000 Americans are diagnosed with melanoma, the deadliest skin cancer. Melanoma is 15 to 20 times more common now than it was 50 years ago, in part, because of depletion of the ozone layer.

Skin cancer is among the most preventable and easily treated of all cancers, yet few doctors perform full skin exams during routine checkups. Insist on it. The vast majority of melanomas can be cured if they're detected and treated at an early stage.

SELF-DEFENSE: At least once a year, ask your primary-care physician or dermatologist to check your entire body for any changes in the size or color of moles or other darkly pigmented areas and/or new growths. Make sure your doctor examines areas that are often missed, such as the scalp, soles of the feet and genitals.

SMART IDEA: Ask your doctor to take pictures of suspicious spots that should be watched. The pictures will provide a baseline comparison for future checkups.

3. *Settling for sigmoidoscopy.* Colon cancer also is among the most treatable of cancers when it's detected early, yet nearly 48,000 Americans die from it needlessly each year.

Unfortunately, many doctors continue to recommend flexible sigmoidoscopy as the only necessary procedure. This test—in which a lighted, hollow tube is inserted through the rectum—

views only the lower half of the colon. Cancers or precancerous polyps present in the upper half of the colon are missed entirely by the procedure.

Colonoscopy is a better choice because it views the entire colon. A study that compared the two tests found that nearly half of 128 patients with advanced cancers or adenomas (abnormal growths that can develop into cancer) had them in the upper colon only—the area not examined by sigmoidoscopy.

SELF-DEFENSE: Get a colonoscopy every 10 years, starting at age 50. Patients with risk factors (a family history of colon cancer or a diagnosis of inflammatory bowel disease) may be advised to start getting the test as early as age 35 or 40.

4. *Cutting good dietary fat.* Most Americans have reduced their intake of dietary fat, both for weight control and disease prevention. Studies show that a low-fat diet reduces the risk for a variety of cancers, including malignancies of the colon and prostate.

The saturated fat from animal sources, such as butter and red meat, does appear to elevate cancer risk. But the monounsaturated fats in many nuts, as well as in olive and canola oils, and the omega-3 fatty acids in such cold-water fish as salmon and tuna appear to have anti-cancer effects. They inhibit the body's production of certain inflammatory *prostaglandins,* natural chemicals that can damage cells and initiate changes that lead to cancer.

A study of more than 6,000 Swedish male twins, recently published in the medical journal *The Lancet,* found that men who did not eat fish were two to three times more likely to get prostate cancer than those who ate fish several times a week. Women who consume large amounts of olive oil may reduce their risk for ovarian cancer by 30%. There's also evidence that olive oil, as well as canola oil, lowers breast cancer risk.

SELF-DEFENSE: Limit all dietary fat to 30% or less of total daily calories...use olive or canola oil to replace butter or vegetable oils (which contain less-healthful polyunsaturated fat)...and substitute several weekly servings of fish for red meat or other foods high in saturated fat.

5. *Drinking too much alcohol.* Although it's true that death rates from cardiovascular disease are lower among men and women who drink moderately than among nondrinkers, the benefits are lost with excessive drinking. In fact, the death rates from cancers of the mouth, esophagus, larynx and liver in men and women who consume at least four drinks daily are three to seven times higher than among nondrinkers. Women who drink more than one drink a day are at increased risk for breast cancer.

SELF-DEFENSE: Men should consume no more than two drinks daily—women, no more than one. If you have a family history or another risk factor for breast cancer, it's probably best to forgo a daily drink.

6. Getting "safe" tans. Most Americans know that excessive sun exposure increases the risk for skin cancer, but some still believe that tanning beds are a safe alternative. Not true. People who use tanning beds are 2.5 times more likely to develop squamous cell carcinoma (in the main structural cells of the epidermis) and 1.5 times more likely to get basal cell carcinoma (in the cells at the lowest layer of the epidermis) than those who don't use them. Some tanning salon sessions expose the body to the same amount of harmful ultraviolet A (UVA) radiation as an entire day at the beach.

SELF-DEFENSE: If you still want a tan, try self-tanners, such as those sold in most drugstores.

■

MEDICAL TESTS THAT CAN SAVE YOUR LIFE

Source: **David Johnson, PhD,** associate professor and chairman in the department of physiology at the University of New England College of Osteopathic Medicine, Biddeford, ME. He is coauthor of *Medical Tests That Can Save Your Life: 21 Tests Your Doctor Won't Order...Unless You Know to Ask.* Rodale.

Many of the most serious medical conditions cause detectable changes in the body long before symptoms appear. Treating health problems at this stage could potentially save thousands of lives every year.

PROBLEM: Doctors rarely look for diseases unless patients have symptoms.

EXAMPLE: An early-stage lung malignancy too small to be seen on a chest X-ray usually causes no symptoms but can be detected by a sophisticated imaging test, known as a low-dose spiral computed tomography (CT) scan. However, few doctors order the test unless patients are coughing up blood, have shortness of breath or other symptoms that indicate an advanced—and far less treatable—stage of lung cancer.

RELUCTANCE TO TEST...

It's impractical to test every person for every possible disease. That's why patients must know their personal risk factors for specific diseases.

Few insurance companies will pay for medical tests in the absence of specific symptoms. But if you have a strong family history of the disease in question, ask your doctor if that justifies testing before symptoms appear.

EXAMPLE: Most insurance companies will not pay for a colonoscopy in people under age 50 but will pay if the test is recommended due to a strong family history of colon cancer.

Serious conditions—and tests to discuss with your doctor...

ANEURYSM...

For various reasons, a bulge can develop in the descending aorta, the main blood vessel from the heart that supplies blood to the legs and organs in the abdomen.

Abdominal aortic aneurysm (AAA) can occur in either men or women but is most common among men ages 50 to 80. Family history (a first-degree relative—parent, sibling or child—who had an aneurysm) increases risk by 12% to 19%.

If the aneurysm ruptures, it causes massive internal bleeding and death in more than 80% of cases. When detected early and treated with surgery, more than 95% of patients are cured.

KEY TEST: An abdominal ultrasound can accurately detect an AAA. During the 10-minute procedure, a technician applies gel to the patient's abdomen and moves a handheld, computerized wand over the area. Abdominal ultrasound measures and records the diameter of the aorta. It can detect a dangerous AAA more than 80% of the time if one is present.

WHO SHOULD CONSIDER TESTING: Anyone with a family history of AAA (ideally, when you are 10 years younger than the age at which your family member was diagnosed)...smokers or former smokers, especially men, with a "pack history" of more than 20 years (one pack a day for 20 years, two packs a day for 10 years, a half pack a day for 40 years, etc.)...and/or anyone with chronic uncontrolled hypertension.

TYPICAL COST: $150.*

CAUTION: Doctors often rely on abdominal palpation and auscultation (listening to arterial sounds through a stethoscope) to detect AAA. These tests are *not* as reliable as abdominal ultrasound.

CAROTID ARTERY DISEASE...

Just like the coronary arteries in the heart, the large neck (carotid) arteries that carry blood to the head and brain can develop atherosclerosis—a buildup of plaque that obstructs circulation and/or promotes the formation of clots.

The first symptom of carotid artery disease (CAD) is often a stroke. Each year, 90,000 Americans have a first or recurrent stroke caused by CAD.

KEY TEST: Duplex ultrasound provides two-dimensional images of the carotid arteries and measures blood flow. It's quick, painless and extremely effective at detecting CAD, particularly in patients with blockages of greater than 70%.

Early detection can greatly reduce the risk for stroke when patients take the appropriate lifestyle and medical steps, such as losing weight...taking cholesterol-lowering or blood pressure medication or a baby aspirin daily...and/or quitting smoking.

WHO SHOULD CONSIDER TESTING: Smokers or former smokers with a 20-year or greater pack history...heavy drinkers (more than three drinks a day)...people who have high cholesterol, elevated triglycerides (a type of blood fat) and/or diabetes...chronic uncontrolled high blood pressure...a first-degree relative with CAD...and/or are obese. African-Americans and people with a family history of heart disease also are at above-average risk for CAD.

TYPICAL COST: $200.*

ADDITIONAL TESTING: If the results of a duplex ultrasound indicate CAD that is severe enough to significantly block blood flow to the head, the doctor will likely order cerebral angiography (a test in which a contrast dye is injected to image the blood vessels of the brain and the flow of blood through them) to confirm the extent of the blockage and whether surgery is necessary.

*Costs are subject to change.

LUNG CANCER...

This is the deadliest cancer because it has usually already spread at the time of diagnosis. The five-year survival rate for most lung cancers is about 16%. However, if detected when the cancer is still localized in the lung, the five-year survival rate is as high as 83%.

KEY TEST: A low-dose spiral CT scan—a painless procedure in which an imaging machine rotates rapidly around the body, taking more than 100 pictures in sequence.

One study found that conventional chest X-rays failed to find 85% of early-stage lung cancers that were detected by low-dose spiral CT.

WHO SHOULD CONSIDER TESTING: Smokers or former smokers with a pack history of 20 years or greater.

TYPICAL COST: $300 to $500.*

PHYSICIANS CAN'T PROTECT YOU FROM SUPERBUGS

Source: **Jerome O. Klein, MD,** professor of pediatrics and vice chairman for academic affairs in the department of pediatrics at Boston University School of Medicine/Boston Medical Center. He is a lecturer at Harvard Medical School, and author of more than 450 articles on infectious diseases.

New strains of drug-resistant bacteria, known as "superbugs," now are being reported with alarming frequency, according to numerous studies.

This is a serious problem. These bacteria are responsible for an increasing number of infections, including pneumonia, sinusitis and ear infections. In fact, bacteria that once responded to antibiotics now are resistant to one or more of these infection-fighting medications.

EXAMPLE: The *Staphylococcus aureus* bacterium, known as staph, is among the most common causes of infection. About *half* of the staph found in intensive-care units can't be killed with the main form of treatment—penicillin-like antibiotics.

*Costs are subject to change.

Drug-resistant forms of staph can cause runaway infections that can't be treated with these standard drugs.

With few new antibiotics in the development pipeline, doctors now worry that even potent antibiotics, such as *vancomycin* (Vancocin), soon will be rendered ineffective.

Here's what you need to know to protect yourself and your family from superbugs...

HOW RESISTANCE DEVELOPS...

When a patient takes an effective antibiotic, the drug kills most of the infection-causing bacteria. A few organisms may survive because they have developed characteristics that make them resistant to the drug. Because the other bacteria have been eradicated, these organisms become the majority. When they multiply, they can create the superbug bacteria that don't respond to previously effective drugs.

These superbugs are transmitted to other people the same way all bacteria are transmitted, through physical contact or droplets spread in the air by coughing or sneezing.

Because bacteria multiply and mutate far more quickly than scientists can develop new antibiotics, there may be fewer available treatments for common—and potentially life-threatening—infections. Patients stay sick longer, and the risk for complications rises.

Antibiotic dangers—and solutions...

DANGER: Taking antibiotics for viral infections.

Most people know that antibiotics treat only infections caused by bacteria and have no effect on viruses. Bacteria have more chances to develop resistance when antibiotics are used more frequently than they should be. Most doctors and patients now recognize the danger.

EXAMPLE: There has been about a 25% decrease in antibiotic prescriptions for respiratory infections since 1995.

HOWEVER: Doctors still write about 50 million unnecessary antibiotic prescriptions annually. Patients who insist that they be given antibiotics for an illness usually get them.

SELF-DEFENSE: Only take antibiotics if your doctor is reasonably sure that the infection is caused by bacteria. The symptoms of viral and bacterial infections are difficult to distinguish, but you probably *don't* need antibiotics if you have a cold or flu.

DANGER: Prescription errors.

Doctors and pharmacists occasionally do make mistakes. A doctor may prescribe the wrong drug or the wrong dose. The pharmacist may misread the instructions.

Taking the wrong antibiotic or the wrong dose can result in a prolonged or untreated infection.

SELF-DEFENSE: Ask your doctor to explain what the drug does before you leave his/her office. Ask what the dose is...how often you're supposed to take it...and for how long.

Then, when you get the prescription filled, check all the information included with the drug. Make sure it corresponds to what your doctor told you.

DANGER: Failing to follow instructions.

Patients often fail to take antibiotics appropriately. They forget doses...or take too much or too little.

SELF-DEFENSE: When you pick up a prescription, read the label instructions before you leave the pharmacy. Ask the pharmacist to clarify information that's unclear.

If the name of the drug is different from what your doctor prescribed, the pharmacist may have substituted the lower-priced generic form of the drug.

DANGER: Being unaware of drug interactions.

Antibiotics, like all medications, can interact with other drugs patients may be taking.

Some antibiotics are best absorbed when taken with meals. Others should be taken on an empty stomach—one hour before or two hours after meals.

Herbs and supplements—calcium supplements, in particular—can inhibit absorption of some antibiotics.

SELF-DEFENSE: Ask your pharmacist if the antibiotic you were prescribed will interact with any medications you are currently taking. Also ask your pharmacist whether the drug should be taken on a full or an empty stomach.

Tell him about any supplements or herbs you are taking, and ask if they will interact with the antibiotic.

DANGER: Stopping treatment early.

Most antibiotics resolve symptoms within a couple of days of treatment. However, some organisms may survive much longer. Patients who quit taking the drugs early—when their symptoms subside—give the hardy survivors a chance to multiply and trigger a new infection that can be harder to treat.

SELF-DEFENSE: Continue taking antibiotics for the full number of days prescribed.

Many antibiotics cause mild side effects, such as nausea or diarrhea. If you experience serious side effects, such as severe diarrhea or hives, call your doctor. If necessary, he can substitute a drug that's less likely to cause serious side effects.

DANGER: Stockpiling.

Patients frequently save unused antibiotics so they can take them at some future time. This is dangerous for the following two reasons.

First, patients who have leftover antibiotics may not have taken the full prescription in the first place. This makes them vulnerable to repeat infections.

Second, antibiotics that were prescribed for one condition may not work for a subsequent illness, even if the symptoms seem similar. In addition, even if the condition is the same, taking a partial dose is unlikely to eradicate infection-causing bacteria.

SELF-DEFENSE: Never save antibiotics. Take the full prescription as prescribed. If your doctor tells you to stop the antibiotic because it is not working, you are experiencing side effects or for some other reason, throw out any remaining pills.

DANGER: Switching drugs unnecessarily.

Doctors treating infections sometimes prescribe a different drug if the first one doesn't seem to be working. This is appropriate in some cases, but switching to a different antibiotic may not always be useful.

SELF-DEFENSE: Ask your doctor how many days it should take for the antibiotic to alleviate symptoms. If you do not experience relief in that amount of time—usually two to three days—alert your doctor.

If your doctor suggests you change antibiotics, find out why. Ask what type of organism is being treated...whether the initial diagnosis was correct...and why the new drug will be more effective than the old one.

■

HOW TO TALK SO DOCTORS WILL LISTEN

Source: **Howard Bruce Beckman, MD,** professor of medicine and family medicine at the University of Rochester School of Medicine and Dentistry in Rochester, NY. He has written more than 50 articles and book chapters on patient–physician communication.

On average, doctor's appointments last just 15 minutes. How do most patients use the time? If they're fortunate, they convey their basic medical complaints and get the bulk of their questions answered in language they can understand. But even well-informed medical consumers often leave a doctor's office unsure of some crucial detail regarding diagnosis or treatment.

To find out how patients can avoid this all-too-common trap, we spoke with Howard Bruce Beckman, MD, a leading authority on doctor–patient communication. **HIS ADVICE...**

• *Make a list.* You may have heard this before, but it really does help. Unfortunately, few patients take the time to do it. Before your appointment, think carefully about the topics you want to discuss and what you hope to get from the visit. Write down your symptoms, the length of time you've experienced them and any other details that you think are relevant. Prioritize the list to ensure that your most important topics get discussed.

• *Set an agenda.* Take a few minutes at the beginning of your appointment to review how the time will be used. The average patient presents three medical concerns during a doctor's appointment. If you don't clarify up front what you hope to gain from your visit, important points are likely to be missed. You have your concerns, but the doctor also may have things he/she wants to bring up. Tell the doctor what you want the visit to accomplish, and ask him if he agrees. For example, you might say, *What I would like to do today is review my test results and then tell you about my shoulder pain. Is that okay?* If you have been explicit and the doctor just ignores you, I suggest you find a new doctor.

• *Be direct.* Some patients are uncomfortable talking about themselves or afraid of bad news, so their communication becomes indirect and/or imprecise. They may even want their doctors to ask them, *What is it that you think you have?* A good doctor will notice if a patient talks about, say, a parent who had a brain tumor. But doctors don't always pick up on these clues.

It is much more effective simply to say, *I keep having these headaches, and I'm worried that it might be a brain tumor.*

• **Find out what to expect from a referral.** If your doctor refers you to a specialist, ask, *What do I have to do to prepare for my visit? What should I expect?* Specialists get advance information from referring physicians only 10% to 20% of the time, so it's important that a patient be prepared to describe his problem to the expert.

Ask your doctor what the specialist is like—many are brilliant doctors but arrogant and difficult to talk with. Patients need to know these details. When appropriate, I tell a patient not to engage the specialist in much conversation. I arrange to have findings sent back to me, and I discuss them with the patient.

• **Don't bog down your doctor with information.** Many patients research their medical conditions on the Internet. This is a good way to learn more about your health problem and double-check that your doctor has presented all treatment options. But don't hand your physician pages of printed material during your appointment. If you've read about a treatment or other information that you think should be considered, summarize the content as well as you can in one page.

• **Articulate the reasons behind your requests.** Many people get upset when their doctors deny them tests that they think are necessary. In many cases, these patients don't understand that the test will not reveal the answer they're seeking. A perfect example is a magnetic resonance imaging (MRI) scan for back pain. In my opinion, there are three legitimate reasons to get an MRI—to find cancer, serious infection or a significant structural disease...to determine operability for disk or other anatomical problems...or to banish an unresolvable fear on the part of the patient. If you clearly state why you want a particular test, you may persuade your doctor to order it—or better understand why he won't.

If a patient has extreme back pain and asks for an MRI, the correct answer, medically speaking, is to wait for six weeks before the test. That's because 90% of patients' symptoms improve within that time. In this case, I tell the patient that he probably has a herniated disk and that he will get better within six weeks. But because most insurance plans cover an MRI, the patient may insist on the test. If he can articulate why he thinks it will be useful in treatment—say, he is desperate to know when he can go back to work—I can explain that the MRI will not give us that answer.

On the other hand, not long ago, I had a headache patient who wanted an MRI. She finally told me she had gotten amoebic dysentery 20 years earlier when she served in the Peace Corps in Sri Lanka. The doctor she saw then predicted she would eventually get an amoebic brain abscess.

I spoke to an infectious disease expert who told me there was no way to be sure her headaches were not related to a brain abscess, so I ordered an MRI. There was no brain abscess, and the patient's headaches resolved after her fears were put to rest.

• *Pinpoint the cause of any disagreement.* A wise professor once taught that if they're arguing about treatment, the doctor and the patient don't agree on the diagnosis. If they're arguing about the diagnosis, they don't agree on the historical facts and the examination results. If you and your doctor disagree on what to do next, take a few steps back and figure out why. Do you think he missed something during the exam? Ignored a symptom? Then have an honest discussion about what needs to be done.

• *Voice your complaints.* Few patients ever give us doctors feedback. They may complain about us in the waiting room and talk to their friends, but they won't confront us directly with what makes them unhappy.

If you are distressed with the way you are treated and feel intimidated about confronting a doctor in person, write a note. Give the doctor a chance to make things right. If your doctor is unresponsive, write a letter to your insurance company or to the physician's practice group. Complaint letters do get read. If you frame the letter as a suggestion for improvement, it most likely will be accepted without defensiveness.

• *Summarize your visit.* Conclude a doctor's appointment by restating what you understand should happen next. Review screening tests that need to be ordered, medications prescribed and lifestyle changes that you have agreed to implement.

If you take the initiative to recap the findings and conclusions of the visit, it often helps the doctor remember something as well. This approach goes a long way toward preventing misunderstandings.

THE AMAZING NO SWEAT EXERCISE PLAN

Source: **Harvey B. Simon, MD,** associate professor of medicine at Harvard Medical School and a founding member of the Harvard Cardiovascular Health Center, both in Boston. Dr. Simon is the author of five previous books on health and fitness. His latest is *The No Sweat Exercise Plan.* McGraw-Hill.

For the past two decades, as "no pain, no gain" has reigned as a fitness mantra, most experts have told us that physical activity won't significantly improve our health unless we perform intense aerobic exercise. It turns out that this was only half the story. Moderate and gentle exercise—everything from sex to yard work—also can help guard against serious illness.

RESEARCHERS IDENTIFY BENEFITS...

Since 2000, more than 22 studies, involving about 320,000 people, have examined how moderate exercise affects health and longevity. The results are stunning. Moderate physical activity can decrease the risks for heart disease (up to 84%)... stroke (up to 34%)...diabetes (up to 50%)...colon malignancies (up to 40%)...and dementia (up to 50%).

When researchers began investigating measures of good health based on everyday activities, they found that even small doses of moderate exercise really do add up. The point is to just get moving. In one study, healthy 20-year-old men were asked to spend three weeks in bed. They developed many physiological characteristics of men twice their age. The same group of men then worked out regularly for eight weeks. They experienced an improvement in weight, resting heart rate, and blood pressure.

HOW TO MEASURE EXERTION...

I felt that a system was needed to measure the value of various everyday physical activities. That's why I created cardiometabolic exercise (CME) points, which assign values to physical activities. You can significantly improve your health by accruing a total of 150 CME points per day (or about 1,000 CME points per week).

IMPORTANT: If weight loss is your goal, you may need to work harder or longer, doubling the target number of CME points to approximately 2,000 per week.

CAUTION: Before starting a new exercise program, consult your doctor. If you have heart disease or are at risk (due to family history, high blood pressure, etc.), you should have a stress test. For healthy people, this simple 12-minute self-test devised by Kenneth H. Cooper, MD, a renowned fitness expert, can help assess your level of fitness. See how far you can go by comfortably walking, jogging or running for 12 minutes (use a pedometer). Your fitness level is considered poor to fair if you cover less than ¾ of a mile…good if you can cover ¾ to one mile…very good for 1 to 1¼ miles…and excellent for more than 1¼ miles.

CREATING A PROGRAM…

For people who use everyday physical activity as the core of their exercise program, it's a good idea to add some strength exercise, such as weight training…some flexibility exercises, such as yoga or stretching…and balance exercises, such as tai chi. Strength training improves muscle mass and bone density. Flexibility exercises help prevent injury and reduce stress. Balance exercises help protect you from falls.

Work up to 20 minutes of strength training two to three times a week…flexibility exercises for 15 minutes three to four times a week…and balance exercises for five minutes three to four times a week.

FITNESS POINTS FOR PHYSICAL ACTIVITIES…

These point values are based on a moderate level of exertion for 30 minutes, unless noted otherwise.

ACTIVITY	CME POINTS	ACTIVITY	CME POINTS
Swimming	230	Walking	125
Aerobics	200	Vacuuming	115
Jogging (12-minute mile)	200	Bowling	100
Mowing lawn		Walking up stairs	
(pushing hand mower)	200	(10 minutes)	100
Tennis (singles)	200	Washing car by hand	100
Golfing (carrying clubs)	165	Cooking	60
Ballroom dancing	150	Washing dishes	60
Gardening	150	Laundering or ironing	
Mowing lawn		(15 minutes)	35
(pushing power mower)	145	Walking down stairs	
Raking leaves	130	(10 minutes)	30
Yoga	130	Sexual activity (15 minutes)	25

Source: The No Sweat Exercise Plan (McGraw-Hill).

■

3

AVOID
MEDICATION
MISHAPS

ASK YOUR DOCTOR TO REVIEW
YOUR MEDICATIONS

Source: **Mark Stengler, ND,** associate clinical professor of family medicine at the National College of Naturopathic Medicine, Portland, OR. He is director of La Jolla Whole Health Clinic, La Jolla, CA, and author of numerous books, including *The Natural Physician's Healing Therapies*. Bottom Line Books.

Ask your doctor to review *all* the medicines you're taking. Even drugs that are thought to be safe may turn out to cause serious side effects. That was the case with *rofecoxib* (Vioxx), the popular analgesic that was recently confirmed to double patients' risk for heart attack. Virtually all drugs cause side effects in some patients, especially in those taking multiple medications.

HELPFUL: Consult with a naturopathic physician. Ask if there are safer alternatives to drug therapy. For example, the supplement policosanol (available at health-food stores) can lower LDL "bad" cholesterol by 15% to 25%. That's comparable with some prescription statins, and policosanol doesn't cause side effects. To find a naturopath in your area, contact the American Association of Naturopathic Physicians, 866-538-2267, *www.naturopathic.org.*

■

PROTECT YOURSELF FROM COX-2s

Source: **Mark Stengler, ND,** associate clinical professor of family medicine at the National College of Naturopathic Medicine, Portland, OR. He is director of La Jolla Whole Health Clinic, La Jolla, CA, and author of numerous books, including *The Natural Physician's Healing Therapies.* Bottom Line Books.

The natural pain reliever methylsulfonylmethane (MSM) is a good substitute for the prescription arthritis drug *celecoxib* (Celebrex) and the over-the-counter painkiller *naproxen* (Aleve). New studies report that these medications may increase heart attack and stroke risk. MSM, a natural compound found in green vegetables, does not cause heart problems or damage the stomach.

TYPICAL DOSE: 2,000 milligrams (mg) twice daily.

CAUTION: Consult your doctor before using MSM if you take a blood thinner. MSM is available at drugstores.

■

DON'T TAKE PRESCRIPTION DRUGS BLINDLY —SOME CAN CAUSE DEPRESSION

Source: **Jack E. Fincham, PhD,** A.W. Jowdy Professor of Pharmacy Care at the University of Georgia, Athens. He is author of *Taking Your Medicine: A Guide to Medication Regimens and Compliance for Patients and Caregivers* (Haworth) and *Troubled Pain Relief: Misused, Overused, and Recalled Analgesic Medications* (Haworth).

Depression is most often caused by a combination of psychological stress and an imbalance in brain chemicals that regulate mood and thought. In some cases, it can have a medical cause, such as an underactive thyroid (hypothyroidism).

HOWEVER: Many prescription and over-the-counter (OTC) drugs also can trigger depression, worsen the condition or interfere with its treatment.

SIDE EFFECTS...

Virtually all drugs can cause side effects, such as headache, upset stomach, sleepiness, nervousness, rash or muscle pain. Many types of medication can also alter mood by directly interfering with the brain chemicals (neurotransmitters) that regulate brain activity.

Individual responses to drugs vary widely, so timing is often a tip-off—depression may begin shortly after you start taking a new drug or increase the dose. Sometimes, it takes longer for your body to respond fully to a drug—the side effect doesn't appear for weeks or more. **DRUGS THAT CAN CAUSE DEPRESSION...**

ANTIBIOTICS...

Almost everyone takes antibiotics from time to time, and side effects, such as upset stomach, come as no surprise. You don't expect a bacteria-killing drug to affect your mood, but insomnia, anxiety—and depression—are possible, especially with certain antibiotics.

This is because these medications disrupt the functioning of neurotransmitters, such as serotonin, acetylcholine and dopamine.

Fluoroquinolones are used widely, especially for upper-respiratory and urinary tract infections. They include *ciprofloxacin* (Cipro), *ofloxacin* (Floxin) and *levofloxacin* (Levaquin). *Metronidazole* (Flagyl) is used to treat bacterial vaginosis.

SOLUTION: If you feel depressed, ask your doctor about switching to an antibiotic from the tetracycline family, such as *doxycycline* (Vibramycin) or *tetracycline* (Achromycin V). The antibiotic *clindamycin* (Cleocin) is an alternative to treat bacterial vaginosis.

Or reducing the dose of metronidazole, the preferred treatment not only for bacterial vaginosis but also for amoebic dysentery, may help.

BLOOD PRESSURE DRUGS...

In some cases, blood pressure medications can lower mood due to their role in depressing the central nervous system

(CNS) or by disrupting the balance of neurotransmitters. Common culprits are the antihypertensives *clonidine* (Catapres) and *methyldopa* (Aldomet) and beta blockers, such as *propranolol* (Inderal) and *atenolol* (Tenormin).

Diuretics, such as *hydrochlorothiazide* (HydroDIURIL), may undermine mood indirectly. Like the other blood pressure drugs listed above, diuretics may interfere with sexual activity, which can lead to depression. Because they stimulate urination, diuretics taken late in the day may disrupt sleep, leading to fatigue and low energy.

SOLUTION: If you feel depressed, ask your doctor about switching to an ACE inhibitor, such as *enalapril* (Vasotec) or *ramipril* (Altace), for blood pressure control. These do not affect the CNS, so they are much less likely to affect mood or sexual function.

HEART FAILURE DRUGS...

Digoxin (Lanoxin), which helps the heart pump more efficiently, is widely used to treat heart failure, and since it affects the CNS, it can cause or worsen depression.

SOLUTION: If you feel depressed, talk to your doctor about using the lowest possible dose of digoxin (typically 0.125 mg) or alternatives, including vasodilators such as *nitroglycerin* (Nitrocot) or *hydrazaline* (Apresoline). An ACE inhibitor, such as *enalapril* (Vasotec), or an angiotensin-receptor blocker (ARB), such as *valsartan* (Diovan), also are alternatives.

HORMONES...

Corticosteroids, such as *prednisolone* (Prelone) and *dexamethasone* (Dexasone), are powerful drugs used to treat a wide variety of conditions, including arthritis, asthma and serious skin problems, such as hives. When taken orally, they can decrease the responsiveness of the CNS, causing profound depression or unnatural euphoria.

SOLUTION: Ask your doctor about reducing the dose, shortening the time that you take the drug or finding an alternative, such as a topical form of the antihistamine *diphenhydramine* (Benadryl) or the OTC antihistamine *loratadine* (Claritin).

IMPORTANT: When used topically or inhaled, corticosteroids are unlikely to affect your mood.

SLEEP AIDS...

These can precipitate mood problems by sapping energy and slowing you down. Benzodiazepines, including tranquilizers such as *alprazolam* (Xanax) and *diazepam* (Valium), often are taken as a sleep aid, but they can cause a next-day "hangover" in susceptible people, including those who are ill.

SOLUTION: Ask your doctor about taking a sleep aid that leaves the body more quickly, such as *zolpidem* (Ambien) or *zaleplon* (Sonata).

OVER-THE-COUNTER DRUGS...

Because OTC medications are available without a prescription, most people don't expect problems. That's a mistake. Although OTC drugs are generally safe if used as directed, they still can cause side effects, including depression.

• *Allergy.* Antihistamines, such as diphenhydramine (Benadryl) and *chlorpheniramine* (Chlor-Trimeton), taken for cold and allergy symptoms, can be extremely sedating (in fact, they're used as OTC sleep aids). These drugs also can lower mood.

SOLUTION: Substitute a nonsedating OTC antihistamine, such as loratadine (Claritin).

• *Heartburn.* Histamine H2 receptor blockers, such as *ranitidine* (Zantac) and *famotidine* (Pepcid), fight heartburn by reducing stomach acid production, but they also affect brain chemicals, which can lead to depression.

SOLUTION: If you feel depressed, replace the H2 blocker with a proton pump inhibitor. It shuts down stomach acid even more completely and does not affect mood. One of these drugs, *omeprazole* (Prilosec), is now available OTC.

■

NEVER IGNORE THESE COMMON SYMPTOMS

DON'T IGNORE THESE DANGEROUS SYMPTOMS...EVEN IF YOUR DOCTOR DOES

Source: **Elaine J. Amella, PhD, APRN,** geriatric nurse practitioner, associate dean for research and evaluation, and associate professor at the College of Nursing, Medical University of South Carolina, Charleston.

Symptoms are the body's way of saying that something is wrong. Crushing chest pain is an urgent warning of possible heart attack...fever and chills signal infection...and excessive thirst and urination may mean diabetes.

However, as we get older, our bodies change—arteries stiffen, kidneys shrink and the immune system slows down. As a result, we not only look and feel different from when we were younger, but we also experience illness differently. That's why it's so important to know the subtle warning signs that mean it's time to see a doctor.

THE CHANGING FACE OF ILLNESS...

There's no set timetable for aging. One person's immune system and circulation may be a lot "younger" at 70 than another's. Aging can be accelerated by chronic conditions (high blood pressure, diabetes, arthritis) or unhealthful lifestyle habits (smoking, drinking alcohol excessively, eating too much and/or exercising too little).

But by the time most people reach 65, their bodies have changed enough that the face of illness may be hard to recognize. Unfortunately, many people dismiss these changes as an unavoidable part of aging.

EXAMPLE: Confusion is *not* natural at any age—nor does it necessarily mean dementia. Possible causes include infection, stress, thyroid disease, vitamin deficiency, dehydration, untreated diabetes and/or adverse effects of medication.

Similarly, aches and pains, dizziness, incontinence, loss of appetite and difficulty performing normal activities, such as shopping and socializing, are frequent indicators of illness and deserve medical attention.

Conditions that cause often-overlooked symptoms...

DEPRESSION...

This mental health problem is as common in older adults as in younger people, and the associated risk for suicide is highest among older white men.

Older adults, however, are less likely to complain of being depressed, while other important symptoms (such as loss of interest in life and troubled sleep) are often dismissed as common signs of advanced age.

TIP-OFF: Physical complaints—headache, muscle pains, stomach upset, fatigue—that have no apparent medical cause are common in depression. The condition also may trigger severe confusion. In older adults, depression is the second most common cause of weight loss (cancer is first).

SELF-DEFENSE: If you feel depressed or experience unexplained physical problems, see your doctor for an evaluation.

HEART ATTACK...

Everyone knows that chest pain is a classic symptom of heart attack. But this symptom—as well as profuse sweating—often does not occur in an older person. If there is pain, it may seem no different from angina (chest pain caused by chronic heart disease).

The landmark Framingham Heart Study found that half of people age 65 or older who had heart attacks between scheduled doctor visits were unaware of them. These "silent" heart attacks were eventually detected via an electrocardiogram (EKG) administered during a checkup.

TIP-OFF: Rapid breathing can occur as the body tries to compensate for lack of oxygen due to failing circulation. Other symptoms include jaw pain, extreme fatigue, confusion and/or severe anxiety. Many people report later that they had an overwhelming sense that something was terribly wrong while the heart attack was going on.

SELF-DEFENSE: If you experience symptoms of a heart attack, call 911.

INFECTION...

We often think of fever as the red flag for infection, but an older person can be quite ill while his/her temperature remains close to normal (98.6°F).

REASON: Fever and chills are caused by chemicals called *cytokines,* which are released by the body's immune system as it fights invading bacteria or a virus. This immune response is known to weaken with age.

ALSO: Body temperature in healthy older adults often is lower than in younger people, probably because of age-related changes in metabolism. What seems "normal" or a very slight fever actually may represent a significant rise.

TIP-OFF: Overall fatigue and a decline in the ability to keep up with the activities of daily life are signs that infection is brewing somewhere in the body. Confusion may be caused by a buildup of toxins released by the pathogen. In some cases, infection may impair nerve and muscle function, leading to falls.

• *Pneumonia* may occur without a cough and/or fever, so it just seems like a bad cold.

TIP-OFF: Breathing becomes unusually rapid (more than 24 breaths per minute) as infected lungs struggle for air. A lack of oxygen may lead to extreme fatigue and an inability to function.

SELF-DEFENSE: If you suffer any symptoms of pneumonia, see your doctor for a diagnosis.

• *Urinary tract infections* can develop in older people without the burning, painful urination that occurs in younger people.

TIP-OFF: Watch for increased frequency of urination...incontinence...confusion...and falls.

SELF-DEFENSE: If you experience any of the symptoms of a urinary tract infection, see your doctor for a urinalysis.

• *Skin infections* are more common in older people, particularly on the legs and feet. Age-related declines in circulation and sensation may mute the pain, leaving you susceptible to an infection and delaying treatment.

TIP-OFF: Be alert for signs of swelling, redness or pus from a wound—even if it doesn't hurt.

SELF-DEFENSE: See your doctor if you experience any symptoms of a skin infection.

THYROID DISEASE...

The two most common symptoms of thyroid disease—fatigue and tremors—may be missing in an older person. Hypothyroidism (underactive thyroid) is most common with aging. Most symptoms of hyperthyroidism (overactive thyroid) are less marked than in younger persons.

TIP-OFF: Muscle weakness, heart palpitations and depression can signal a thyroid problem. Because confusion also can occur, family members may write off an older adult as being demented, when treating the thyroid problem could restore mental function.

SELF-DEFENSE: See your doctor if you suffer from any thyroid disease symptoms. He/she may order a thyroid-stimulating hormone (TSH) test—a blood test to measure thyroid function.

TYPE 2 DIABETES...

Nearly 19% of Americans over age 60 have diabetes. It is the fifth leading cause of death in the US. In older people, diabetes may go unrecognized for years, because the classic symptoms—thirst, excessive urination and increased appetite—are missing.

TIP-OFF: The high blood sugar caused by type 2 diabetes often triggers confusion. Dehydration may lead to decreased urination, a sunken look around the eyes and hot, dry skin. Yeast or fungal infections may occur, or a skin ulcer may not heal. Chronic urinary tract infection, incontinence and weight loss may occur.

SELF-DEFENSE: Everyone should be screened for diabetes with a fasting blood glucose test at age 45 and, if results are normal, every three years thereafter. Those under age 45 should be screened if they have a body mass index (BMI) greater than 25 or other risk factors.*

■

SNORING MAY SIGNAL LARGER PROBLEMS

Source: **David L. Steward, MD,** associate professor and director of the clinical trials program in the department of otolaryngology at the University of Cincinnati College of Medicine and member of the Obstructive Sleep Apnea Committee of the American Academy of Otolaryngology, Alexandria, VA.

U p to 80% of men and 30% of women snore on occasion. Unfortunately, most people dismiss snoring as nothing more than a nuisance. That's a mistake.

Snoring can be a sign of potentially serious health problems.

EXAMPLE: Obese people often snore. So do those with sleep apnea, in which breathing stops periodically during sleep. Both conditions increase the risk for high blood pressure and heart disease.

Anyone whose snoring is loud enough to disturb a bed partner—or is accompanied by morning headaches or daytime fatigue—should be evaluated by an otolaryngologist (ear, nose and throat specialist) who specializes in sleep disorders.**

Main causes of snoring...

SLEEP APNEA...

This condition is defined as a complete or partial breathing blockage occurring more than five times an hour or more than 40 times during eight hours of sleep. Many sleep apnea patients stop breathing hundreds of times per night. The sufferers must arouse themselves from sleep to start breathing

*To determine your BMI, go to *www.nhlbisupport.com/bmi/bmicalc.htm*, or use the formula (weight in pounds x 703) ÷ height in inches squared. A BMI of 25 to 29.9 is considered overweight...30 and above is obese.

**To find a sleep specialist in your area, contact the American Academy of Otolaryngology, 703-836-4444, *www.entnet.org.*

again, which prevents them from getting restful sleep. Studies have shown that patients with sleep apnea may be so fatigued during the day that they have slower reaction times than drunk drivers have.

Sleep apnea is usually caused by excess tissue in the throat that sags and obstructs the flow of air. The condition primarily affects overweight men and women. Men with a neck size of 17 inches or larger have the greatest risk of developing the condition. Both apnea and snoring can be significantly improved when patients lose weight.

A form-fitting mouthpiece, prescribed by a doctor, can help prevent snoring. It pulls the tongue and soft palate forward to keep the airways open. You can read up on a variety of mouthpieces online at an oral appliance Web site, such as Quiet Sleep, *www.quietsleep.com*. If the mouthpiece needs to be used nightly, a custom-made device is most comfortable and will not cause jaw or dental problems. It can be ordered from your dentist or oral surgeon for about $800.

ALSO HELPFUL: Sleep on your side. This position reduces the effect of gravity on tissues in the throat and helps keep the airways open.

Continuous positive airway pressure (CPAP), in which patients wear a pressurized mask during sleep, successfully eliminates apnea and snoring in nearly all patients, but requires nightly use to be effective. With CPAP, air is forced through the airways and prevents them from collapsing.

Until recently, surgery was the only other option. Depending on the patient, this may involve *uvulopalatopharyngoplasty* (removing tissue from the soft palate as well as the uvula), which is usually performed in conjunction with removal of tonsils...removing enlarged adenoids...or tightening throat tissue. In some cases, the upper and/or lower jaw may need reshaping to improve airflow.

NEW APPROACH: Radio frequency therapy (somnoplasty) uses radio waves to shrink the soft palate or other enlarged tissues. The outpatient procedure, performed by an otolaryngologist with local anesthesia, takes about 30 minutes. Patients receive as many as five treatments. It's safer than surgery, since it does not require general anesthesia—which can be risky for obese patients with sleep apnea—and can be used as an alternative to CPAP for serious apnea and snoring.

ALCOHOL...

Drinking depresses the central nervous system, increases relaxation of throat muscles and promotes congestion by dilating blood vessels in the nose. Just one to two drinks can make snoring worse.

It's fine for most people to have a beer or a glass of wine with dinner if snoring is mild—but don't have a nightcap within two hours of bed. People with loud or frequent snoring may want to give up alcohol for a few weeks to see if it helps.

ALLERGIES...

Nasal congestion that accompanies allergies results in mouth-breathing during sleep, which can increase snoring.

If you have itchy, watery eyes as well as congestion, allergies may be the culprit. To determine whether allergies are causing you to snore, use a decongestant nasal spray, such as *oxymetazoline* (Afrin), for a few nights. If the snoring improves, nasal congestion is probably the problem.

CAUTION: Do *not* continue using the spray. Daily use can cause *rebound congestion* that's worse than the original problem.

Avoiding allergens is the best defense.

EXAMPLE: Stay indoors during peak pollen times (in the mornings and evenings)...wash your bedding in hot water weekly to kill dust mites...control mold by wiping damp surfaces with a mild bleach solution...and use a dehumidifier in basements or other damp areas.

Nonsedating oral antihistamines, such as *loratadine* (Claritin), can reduce nasal congestion and snoring. Your doctor may prescribe a nasal steroid spray, such as *fluticasone* (Flonase), to shrink nasal swelling. Intranasal steroid sprays don't cause rebound congestion and are safe for long-term use.

DEVIATED SEPTUM...

The partition between the nostrils is sometimes crooked, usually from birth or due to a broken nose or other trauma. This reduces airflow, which often causes snoring.

Air normally flows through alternate sides of the nose at different times—it switches every four to six hours. If you consistently breathe through only one side of your nose, you may have a deviated septum. Surgery to repair the septum is helpful in severe cases, but most patients simply can use a nasal steroid, such as *triamcinolone* (Nasacort) or *budesonide* (Rhinocort), to reduce swelling and help air to flow more smoothly.

ALSO HELPFUL: Use an over-the-counter nasal strip, such as Breathe Right, to help hold the nasal passages open.

NASAL POLYPS...

These benign growths are usually caused by persistent infections and/or allergies. A polyp no larger than a pencil eraser can obstruct normal airflow and cause snoring.

Polyps usually disappear once nasal inflammation or infection is treated with medication. If they don't go away—or keep coming back—you may need to have them surgically removed in a 30- to 60-minute outpatient procedure that requires general anesthesia.

TURBINATE HYPERTROPHY...

The turbinates are small, bony structures that protrude into the nasal airway. They're covered with a mucous membrane that warms and moisturizes incoming air. Enlarged turbinates, due to allergies, obstruct airflow and often cause snoring.

Radio frequency treatments shrink turbinates and reduce snoring. Most patients need only one treatment to eliminate scar tissue and enlarge the nasal openings.

■

YOUR DOCTOR MAY MISS
THE SIGNS OF DEPRESSION

Source: **Michael E. Thase, MD,** professor of psychiatry at the University of Pittsburgh Medical Center. He is coauthor of *Beating the Blues: New Approaches to Overcoming Dysthymia and Chronic Mild Depression.* Oxford University.

Virtually everyone has occasional moods when life seems dreary and pointless and nothing brings much pleasure or satisfaction. These normally pass, and a few hours or days later, you're feeling fine.

For some people, however, such feelings do *not* pass. They're not so down that they can't work or see friends, but life has lost its sparkle. Although this chronic, low-level depression —known as *dysthymia*—affects about 3 million Americans, it often goes undetected by the sufferers themselves, their families and even their doctors.

Unlike grief—a natural reaction to a death or other loss that gets better over time—dysthymia has no apparent reason and keeps your spirits low for the greater part of most days. Sadness may predominate, or the feeling may be one of apathy, emotional numbness or an inability to enjoy the things you once did.

You can help manage the symptoms of your condition by reevaluating and changing how you *think* and *act*.

YOU CAN CHANGE...

Many scientists believe that chronic depression is linked to a tendency, perhaps inherited, for brain chemicals to get out of balance.

Stress or trauma early in life can also play a role as well as chronic health or personal problems in adulthood. But no matter where it comes from, a major part of the condition is a negative way of thinking that generates unpleasant emotions.

It's normal to think negative thoughts approximately 20% of the time, but for depressed people these thoughts consume more than 70% of their inner monologue.

Changing these patterns can make a difference in how you feel. **HERE'S HOW...**

• *Substitute optimism for pessimism.* The "half-empty glass" outlook condemns you to live in a world where nothing seems likely to work out well.

Pessimistic people tend to *generalize* from unpleasant events, believe distressing circumstances are *permanent* and *personalize* bad experiences. A more realistic view—that most difficulties are limited in scope, temporary and impersonal—can keep you out of the depressive spiral.

EXAMPLE: You're shortchanged by a grocery clerk, who is rude when you call it to her attention. You immediately think, *Everyone is out to cheat me.*

MORE REALISTIC: *This person is just a jerk.*

To combat the negative way of thinking, start monitoring your thoughts. Whenever you find yourself thinking globally and personally, get down to specifics to limit the pain you cause yourself.

EXAMPLE: When your inner voice says, *Nothing goes my way,* try, *This week has really been tough.*

• *Schedule pleasurable activities.* Depression slows you down and saps your energy. It's a vicious cycle—the less you do, the more you think about your problems.

Something as simple as a movie, lunch with a friend, gardening or listening to music can provide a small but real lift to your spirits.

Think of enjoyment as a *prescription.* Plan at least one or two potentially pleasurable activities every day—*even if you're not in the mood.*

HELPFUL: In a journal, rate from one to 10 how much you expect to enjoy a concert, dinner out, massage, etc. Afterward, rate the actual experience. You may get more pleasure than you expected.

• *Make yourself exercise.* It releases endorphins and balances other brain chemicals to reduce tension, frustration and stress...raises your energy level...and distracts your attention from negative thoughts.

WHEN TO GET HELP...

If you've done what you can on your own but still feel down, it's time to seek expert assistance. Both medication and psychotherapy can work quite well for chronic depression.

A good therapist will help you understand how your thinking habits, social skills and relationship difficulties contribute to your depression, and support your concrete steps to change them. Just three months of such therapy can be effective.

The same antidepressant medications used for severe acute depression work with chronic low-level forms as well. Among the most commonly used antidepressants are *sertraline* (Zoloft), *fluoxetine* (Prozac), *bupropion* (Wellbutrin) and *venlafaxine* (Effexor).

Each is effective 50% to 60% of the time, so it may take some trial and error to find the drug that works best for you.

If you're reluctant to try a prescription antidepressant, ask your doctor about taking the herb St. John's wort (900 to 1,200 milligrams [mg] daily for four to six weeks).

■

5 ✚

BEAT THE
MEDICAL SYSTEM

DON'T BECOME A VICTIM
OF MEDICAL NEGLECT

Source: **Pamela F. Gallin, MD,** director and professor, pediatric ophthalmology, Columbia University Medical Center and Columbia University College of Physicians and Surgeons, both in New York City. She has served on the White House Health Care Task Force and is author of *How to Survive Your Doctor's Care.* Lifeline Press.

Even doctors, who know the ins and outs of the health-care system and get better-than-average care, fall victim to medical errors and neglect.

EXAMPLE: Four days after I had hand surgery in 1988, I had incredible pain. The surgeon, thinking I was overreacting, wouldn't even give me an appointment to see him.

I did get in to see one of his colleagues, who immediately took off the cast. It had been put on too tightly and was damaging nerves and impeding circulation. It took six months for the nerves to recover—and worse, I could have lost the use of the hand.

Time pressures, cost-saving measures and the endless maze of insurance bureaucracies all guarantee that mistakes *will* happen. So now it's up to patients to make sure mistakes don't happen to them. **HERE'S HOW...**

CHOOSE THE RIGHT HOSPITAL...

Your primary-care doctor is just one of many who will tend to your care. You want to make sure that *all* of your doctors and nurses are the best available—and the place to find them is usually at a major medical center affiliated with a teaching university.

These hospitals offer the latest and most effective tests and treatments. All of your primary-care doctor's colleagues—radiologists, anesthesiologists, etc.—will have similar levels of training. No matter where you live, there's probably a major teaching hospital within a few hours' drive and affiliates even closer to your home.

CAUTION: Many major medical centers lend their names to suburban hospitals and clinics. Don't assume that they all offer the same level of care. If your doctor serves at one of these affiliates, ask if he/she also has privileges at the main institution.

PICK THE RIGHT KIND OF DOCTOR...

Many patients choose family-practice physicians or obstetrician/gynecologists as their primary-care doctors. That's fine if you're young and healthy, but if you have pre-existing conditions or are age 35 or older, your primary-care physician should be an internist.

Internists tend to know more about evaluating—and treating—diseases and are trained to coordinate your overall care if you need multiple doctors. Many internists have additional training in other specialties, such as rheumatology, cardiology or gastroenterology. Pick an internist whose training matches *your* medical needs.

IMPORTANT: Your doctor should be board-certified in his area of expertise. The Web site *www.docboard.org* offers background information on physicians, including notations on disciplinary actions and medical malpractice lawsuits that have been filed.

QUESTION YOUR DIAGNOSIS...

Two equally competent doctors can look at the same test results and arrive at different conclusions.

Always get a second opinion if you've been diagnosed with a serious health problem, such as cancer or a heart condition.

If the second opinion differs from the first, ask doctor No. 2 why doctor No. 1 is mistaken. Get as much information as you can. Don't hesitate to get even a third opinion if the first two are conflicting.

IMPORTANT: Get the second opinion from a doctor who specializes in your condition.

The sister of a friend of mine was told by her internist that her lung cancer had recurred, based on an abnormal chest X-ray. She got a second opinion from a pulmonary oncologist, who performed several tests, including magnetic resonance imaging (MRI), blood tests and a biopsy. The second doctor determined that the problem was merely inflammation. The internist wasn't a bad doctor. He got it wrong because he wasn't a trained oncologist.

ALWAYS REPEAT "BAD" TESTS...

Diagnostic and treatment errors often are due to faulty tests or an improper interpretation of the results. If a test indicates that you have a serious problem, consider having it repeated. Be especially suspicious when test results that were normal in the past suddenly seem much worse.

IMPORTANT: If your test was done at a small hospital or clinic, have the test results sent to a major medical center for a second opinion. This usually costs $100 to $150, and your insurance may pay for it.

ALSO: Ask that your tests be read by a pathologist or radiologist who specializes in that particular part of the body.

EXAMPLE: If you've had a computed tomography (CT) scan of your head to investigate a possible tumor, the films should be reviewed by a neuroradiologist at a major medical center. A general radiologist who works at a local hospital may misinterpret the findings.

PICK YOUR SURGERY TEAM...

If you need an operation, it's not enough just to choose your surgeon. You also should be involved in picking the anesthesiologist. Anesthesia is one of the most dangerous parts of surgery.

Key points...

• *Ask your surgeon to include an anesthesiologist* who specializes in your condition.

EXAMPLE: A neuroanesthesiologist if you will need to have neurosurgery.

• *Ask for an anesthesiologist who works with your surgeon frequently.* Good teamwork will reduce the risk of complications.

• *Request a board-certified anesthesiologist.* This is especially true if you're having a lengthy or complicated procedure, such as cardiac or abdominal surgery.

■

DON'T COUNT ON YOUR DOCTOR— BE YOUR OWN HEALTH ADVOCATE

Source: **Charles B. Inlander,** a consumer advocate and health-care consultant based in Fogelsville, PA. He is author of more than 20 books on consumer health issues, including *Take This Book to the Hospital with You: A Consumer Guide to Surviving Your Hospital Stay.* St. Martin's.

Having a family member or friend present at doctors' appointments is like having another set of ears to hear what the doctor is saying and a second voice to ask the questions that need to be asked.

Most doctors appreciate an advocate being present, especially if the patient is under great stress or is otherwise unable to comprehend all that's being discussed. Any patient who has a serious health problem or faces a major course of medical treatment would be wise to take someone along on doctors' appointments. When a person's health is at stake, it can be incredibly stressful, which means the patient is probably not operating at 100% of his/her mental capacity.

But just accompanying someone on a doctor's appointment is not enough. **HERE'S HOW TO BE A GOOD ADVOCATE...**

• *Write questions in advance.* To use your time with the doctor most efficiently, divide the questions into two categories. First list the questions that apply directly to the patient, such as *What do you expect to find from this test?* or *Should the medication be taken in the morning or evening?* Then list the questions that involve the advocate or caregiver, such as *Will he need assistance at home after the surgery?*

• *Be sure the patient is included.* Once at the doctor's office, make sure the doctor speaks directly to the patient at all times. Too often, the doctor assumes that the patient won't understand what's being discussed and speaks to the advocate. But even if the patient doesn't understand, he still can hear and probably feels nervous. It's very reassuring when the doctor focuses on the patient. On the other hand, if the doctor ignores the advocate's questions, it may be helpful for the patient to say, *I've brought along my friend (daughter, neighbor, etc.), and I'd like her to be included in all discussions.* During the appointment, the advocate should take notes. If the doctor asks the patient a question, the advocate first should let the patient try to answer. If he cannot, then the advocate can respond, if appropriate. Before leaving, the advocate should verbally review what the doctor has said.

• *Don't forget the office staff.* The advocate should introduce himself to the receptionist and any staffers who assist during the appointment. Be sure also to get the name of the doctor's primary nurse. Ask if it is okay if you call the receptionist or the doctor's nurse directly if you have any follow-up questions or concerns. Ask for the best times to call.

Most important, don't be shy. Remember that you are representing a person who is relying on you for help.

■

DON'T BE DECEIVED BY
DRUG COMPANY TACTICS

Source: **Marcia Angell, MD,** former editor–in–chief of *The New England Journal of Medicine* and now a senior lecturer at Harvard Medical School's department of social medicine in Boston. She is a nationally recognized authority in the field of health policy and medical ethics and an outspoken critic of the health-care system. She is author of *The Truth About Drug Companies: How They Deceive Us and What to Do About It.* Random House.

In light of the recent revelations about the harmfulness of the prescription drug *rofecoxib* (Vioxx) and other painkillers, drug companies have come under increased scrutiny.

FACT: Between 1997 and 2001, drug companies tripled the amount of money they spent on direct-to-consumer advertising for prescription drugs—the ads now seen so frequently on television and in newspapers.* The number of retail prescriptions rose from 2.4 billion in 1997 to 3.1 billion in 2001. Those prescriptions carry a total yearly price tag of at least $200 million, with the cost rising about 12% per year, approximately six times the rate of inflation.

But doesn't the increased use of medications signal better health for Americans? Not necessarily.

To learn more about the claims made by drug companies, we spoke to Marcia Angell, MD, former editor–in–chief of the prestigious *New England Journal of Medicine...*

CLAIM: The increased costs of drugs reflect large investments in research and development (R&D).

FACT: Drug companies spend more than twice as much on "marketing and administration" as they do on R&D—31% of sales, compared with 14% in 2003.

Drug industry sources say the R&D cost per drug is $800 million, on average. An independent analysis by the nonprofit consumer advocacy organization Public Citizen shows that the real cost is probably $100 million or less.

Actually, the big drug companies don't develop most of the novel medications. These drugs, such as the cancer medications *paclitaxel* (Taxol) and *imatinib* (Gleevec), mostly are the result of taxpayer-funded research at academic institutions or the National Institutes of Health (NIH) or research at small biotechnology companies.

CLAIM: New drugs are constantly being brought to market.

FACT: Of the 487 drugs approved by the FDA from 1998 through 2003, only 32% contained new active ingredients and fewer than half of those (14% of the total) were classified by the FDA as improvements over older drugs.

Most "new" drugs are chemical variations of older drugs already on the market—so-called "me-too" drugs. Companies try to grab a piece of a profitable market by producing a medication similar to a top-selling drug.

EXAMPLE: Mevacor, approved in 1987, was the first cholesterol-lowering statin in the marketplace. Now, there are five more, all variants of the original—Lipitor, Zocor, Pravachol,

*2001 is the most recent year for which information is complete.

Lescol and Crestor. Even though Lipitor and Zocor are the top-selling statins, no head-to-head studies have been conducted comparing their effectiveness with *lovastatin* (the cheaper generic form of Mevacor) when taken at equivalent doses.

CLAIM: Scientific studies on drugs are reliable.

FACT: Drug companies have always sponsored almost all research on their drugs, but now they control how the research is done and whether it will be published. Much of this research is seriously flawed, presenting results that cause both doctors and consumers to believe that drugs are a lot better than they are and have fewer side effects than they do. What's more, only favorable results are published. Unfavorable results rarely see the light of day.

CLAIM: Doctors' prescribing habits aren't unduly influenced by drug companies.

FACT: In 2001, the drug industry employed approximately 88,000 sales representatives to visit doctors in their offices and hospitals to promote their products—roughly one representative for every six practicing physicians. Drug reps attend medical conferences and offer doctors expensive gifts. Although some doctors refuse these gifts, many do accept dinners, football tickets, family vacations, etc.

In 2001, drug companies paid more than 60% of the costs for continuing medical education for doctors. Meetings of professional societies, such as the American College of Cardiology and the American College of Physicians, now are largely sponsored by drug companies.

Knowing this, do you think the prescribing habits of doctors in America are based only on the objective evaluations of their patients?

WHAT YOU CAN DO...

To protect yourself against drug industry tactics...

• *Ignore drug ads.* An ad is meant to sell something, not educate or inform. Drug ads are no different. There's a good reason that direct-to-consumer drug ads are illegal in every other developed country (except New Zealand).

• *Be skeptical about new drugs.* When it comes to drugs, newer doesn't necessarily mean better. There are exceptions, but you should make sure your doctor is relying on scientific evidence, not just a sales pitch from a drug company.

- *Watch out for "me-too" drugs.* If a drug is being advertised on TV, it's probably a me-too drug. The drug company is trying to convince doctors and patients—usually in the absence of any scientific evidence—that the "new" drug is better.

- *Always ask for an equivalent generic or over-the-counter (OTC) drug.* Doctors tend to prescribe what the drug company reps who haunt their offices are pushing. There may be a cheaper alternative that's just as effective. Ask about it.

- *Beware of free samples.* Drug reps give doctors free samples of expensive drugs. When the sample runs out, both doctor and patient are in the habit of using that particular drug. If you accept a free sample, be sure there is a compelling medical reason to take that drug.

- *Don't be easily convinced that you have a new disease.* Do you really need to take the me-too antidepressant *paroxetine* (Paxil) for "social anxiety disorder"—when you thought you were just shy?

- *Give your doctor permission not to prescribe.* Many doctors assume—correctly, in many cases—that a patient won't feel satisfied unless he/she leaves the office with a prescription.

TELL YOUR MD: *If I don't need a prescription drug, then don't prescribe one.*

■

WHAT YOUR LAB TESTS REALLY MEAN

Source: **Kandice Kottke-Marchant, MD, PhD,** chair, division of pathology and laboratory medicine, The Cleveland Clinic, and professor and chairperson, department of pathology at the Cleveland Clinic Lerner College of Medicine of Case Western Reserve University.

Even if they're health-savvy, few patients know as much as they should about diagnostic blood and urine tests.

RESULT: Patients are less able to help spot errors that could lead to a physician's misdiagnosis and/or inappropriate treatment. **KEY FACTS...**

LABORATORY TESTS...

The complete blood count (CBC) measures the number of cells in your blood. Hundreds of diseases can cause abnormalities in these counts, including infections, some cancers and blood disorders.

Urinalysis evaluates the appearance and chemistry of your urine. Abnormalities can signal kidney disease, urinary tract infections, some types of cancer or diabetes.

You should review your lab reports with your physician. Keep a copy of each report in your files to compare it with past or future results. Printouts include a "reference range," the statistically normal values for a person your age.

WHAT MOST PEOPLE DON'T KNOW: Some people are what pathologists call "outliers"—that is, even though healthy, they have slightly higher or lower values in one or more categories. Further testing typically is required.

INTERPRETING THE CBC...

A CBC may be ordered prior to surgery and/or for evaluation of an infection, fatigue, fever, anemia, cancer or heart disease. The CBC analyzes white blood cells (WBCs), red blood cells (RBCs) and platelets, all of which are produced in the bone marrow.

Most important measurements...

• *WBC count.* WBCs battle viruses, bacteria and other infectious agents. They are measured in thousands per cubic millimeter (K/mm^3) of blood.

NORMAL RANGE: 4.0 to 11.0.*

• *WBC differential.* This measures the relative percentage of five types of WBCs—neutrophils (which fight bacterial infection)...basophils and eosinophils (they play a role in allergic responses)...and lymphocytes and monocytes (which develop in an immune response to many infections). Ask your doctor for your normal ranges.

• *Absolute neutrophil count (ANC).* This uses a formula involving "polys" (mature neutrophils) and "bands" (young neutrophils). A decreased ANC can signal bone marrow failure, while a high ANC is seen with infections and some leukemias.

NORMAL RANGE: 38% to 78% of all WBCs.

*Normal ranges vary slightly from lab to lab.

WHAT YOUR RESULTS MAY MEAN: Problems with WBCs could signal an infection...a disorder of the bone marrow...or just an allergy.

• *RBC count.* RBCs carry oxygen to, and remove carbon dioxide from, the tissues. They are measured in millions per cubic millimeter (mil/mm³) of blood.

NORMAL RANGE: 4.5 to 6 for men...4.2 to 5.4 for women.

• *Hemoglobin (HGB) value.* Hemoglobin is the protein that carries oxygen, and it is measured in grams per deciliter (g/dl) of blood.

NORMAL RANGE: 13.5 to 17.5 for men...12 to 16 for women.

• *Hematocrit (HCT) value.* HCT is the percentage of your blood that consists of RBCs. A decrease in HCT indicates anemia, which can result in too little oxygen being delivered to the tissues.

NORMAL RANGE: 40% to 52% for men...37% to 47% for women.

WHAT YOUR RESULTS MAY MEAN: Problems with RBCs are a sign of anemia, bleeding, some cancers, bone marrow disease or a drug side effect, typically from chemotherapy.

• *Platelet count.* Platelets form clots and stop bleeding. They're measured in thousands per cubic millimeter (K/mm³) of blood.

NORMAL RANGE: 150 to 400.

WHAT YOUR RESULTS MAY MEAN: Problems with platelets can signal leukemia, thrombocytopenia (too few platelets), rare congenital disorders or a drug side effect.

INTERPRETING URINALYSIS...

If you complain of low back pain, painful or frequent urination, or discover that you have dark or bloody urine, your physician should order a urinalysis.

Most important components...

• *Protein.* Normally, the kidneys do not allow protein to leak into the urine. The presence of high levels—above 10 mg/100 ml—suggests an abnormality, such as kidney disease. If a high protein level is found, other kidney function tests, such as creatinine, should be ordered.

• *Glucose and ketones.* Excess levels indicate diabetes. If you have high glucose or ketones, your doctor should order a blood glucose test and other diabetes screening tests, such as hemoglobin A1C.

- **Nitrite.** High levels of this compound indicate a urinary tract infection.
- **Leukocyte esterase.** When present in the urine, this enzyme (produced by white blood cells) may indicate an infection.
- **Casts.** The presence of casts (cellular deposits formed in the kidney), and their specific type, can indicate many problems, including kidney disease and diabetes.
- **Crystals.** When present in small numbers, most crystals, such as those made of calcium oxalate, are not significant. Others, such as crystals of the amino acid *leucine,* can indicate severe liver disease.
- **RBCs.** High levels of RBCs can indicate trauma to the kidney or urinary tract, cancer or urinary tract infections.

PREVENTING ERRORS...

The automated instruments that analyze blood are precise, and most CBCs are accurate. Similarly, few mistakes are made with a typical urinalysis, but errors can occur.

Best ways to avoid lab errors...

- **Make sure your doctor or hospital uses an accredited lab.** Yearly inspections are required for labs accredited by organizations such as the College of American Pathologists. To find out if a lab is accredited, ask the lab or hospital administrator.
- **Don't assume that your tube is labeled correctly.** Mix-ups can occur. Ask the lab technician, *How did you label the tube?*

EVEN BETTER: Ask politely to see the tube, so you're sure it has your name on it.

- **Check for clots.** If blood takes more than two minutes to fill the tube, it will likely clot in the process. This renders it useless for a CBC. Ask the lab technician, *Does my tube have any clots in it?*

EVEN BETTER: Ask to see the tube, and tilt it gently. If there's a large clot, you'll see it.

■

6

BEWARE OF
MEDICAL MYTHS

DANGEROUS MEDICAL MYTHS

Sources: **Michael F. Roizen, MD,** chair of the division of anesthesiology, critical care medicine and comprehensive pain management at the Cleveland Clinic, and **Mehmet C. Oz, MD,** director of the Cardiovascular Institute at Columbia University Medical Center in New York City. Dr. Roizen and Dr. Oz are coauthors of *You: The Owner's Manual.* HarperCollins.

Most people unintentionally increase their risk for illness, premature aging and even death simply because they lack key facts about their own bodies.

PROBLEM: Because doctors don't have time to educate patients about everything that could possibly go wrong with their health, you need to have a basic understanding of what kinds of symptoms to watch for...and which medical advice can be trusted.

Some of the most common beliefs are the most dangerous...

MYTH: Ulcers aren't contagious. Nearly all ulcers are caused by *Helicobacter pylori* (H. pylori), a spiral-shaped bacterium that penetrates the stomach lining. A blood test can detect H. pylori in people with ulcer symptoms, including pain in the abdominal area just above the navel. Doctors can successfully eradicate H. pylori with a two-week course of antibiotics, but the ulcers frequently return.

REASON: Kissing can transmit the bacterium. Even if an ulcer patient is successfully treated with antibiotics, he/she can reacquire the bacterium—and the ulcer—from H. pylori-infected saliva.

RECOMMENDATION: If you or your spouse or partner has ulcers due to H. pylori, ask your doctor about *both* of you taking antibiotics to avoid reinfecting one another. Also, get a new toothbrush to avoid reinfecting yourself.

MYTH: High blood pressure begins at 140/90. Until recently, doctors didn't consider blood pressure to be elevated unless it was above 140/90. According to the National Heart, Lung, and Blood Institute, a patient who has a blood pressure reading as low as 120/80 has *prehypertension*—and is at an increased risk for heart disease.

Optimal blood pressure is 115/76. The difference of just a few points might seem insignificant, but patients who maintain blood pressure readings at this level or lower have *half* the cardiovascular risk of those at the higher level.

RECOMMENDATION: Because many doctors don't flag blood pressure readings that are only slightly elevated, ask the nurse/ technician taking your blood pressure what your reading is. If it is above 115/76, ask your doctor how to bring it down.

Slight elevations can almost always be controlled with lifestyle changes, such as losing just five to 10 pounds, exercising and increasing fruit and vegetable intake.

MYTH: If your cholesterol levels are normal, you won't have a heart attack. Most heart attack sufferers have normal cholesterol levels.

Few people realize that heart attacks are typically caused by blood clots that form on top of irritated, inflamed areas of plaque (a mixture of cholesterol and other substances) on artery walls. When these clots grow, they can lodge in an artery and cause a heart attack.

Lowering low-density lipoprotein (LDL or "bad") cholesterol creates a less favorable environment for clot formation. If your doctor says your LDL cholesterol is elevated, implement lifestyle changes, such as diet and exercise.

Still, some researchers speculate that statins, such as *atorvastatin* (Lipitor), work not so much by lowering cholesterol but rather by reducing the arterial inflammation that promotes blood clots.

In fact, studies have shown that statins reduce heart attack risk even in patients with normal cholesterol levels.

IMPORTANT: Do *not* take more than 100 milligrams (mg) of vitamin C or 100 international units (IU) of vitamin E daily if you are also taking a statin. These vitamins inhibit the drug's anti-inflammatory effects.

In addition to statins, there are other effective strategies to help prevent inflammation and clots.

RECOMMENDATION 1: Care for your teeth. Brush *and* floss daily. Get a professional cleaning twice a year.

The bacteria that cause gum disease also can promote inflammation and plaque in the arteries.

RECOMMENDATION 2: Consider aspirin therapy. Ask your doctor about taking two 81-mg "baby" (or half an adult) aspirin daily to reduce arterial inflammation and inhibit clots.

HELPFUL: Buy regular, cheap aspirin. Drink one-half glass of water before and after taking the aspirin. This helps in the absorption and makes the aspirin less likely to cause gastrointestinal bleeding.

IMPORTANT: Some recent studies have questioned whether aspirin really does help prevent heart disease, but we recommend this therapy for patients who are candidates because it also helps curb the risk for colon, breast, prostate and other types of cancers.

MYTH: **Fiber prevents colon cancer.** Eating fruits and vegetables can help prevent colon malignancies and other cancers, but research shows that it isn't the fiber in these foods that does the trick—it's the antioxidants.

Although there are many reasons to get plenty of dietary fiber—for example, it prevents constipation, improves digestion and helps lower LDL cholesterol levels—studies have shown that other approaches are more effective at preventing colon cancer.

RECOMMENDATION 1: Ask about aspirin. Two baby (or half an adult) aspirin daily reduces your risk for colon cancer by 40%, possibly due to its anti-inflammatory effect. Ask your doctor if aspirin is right for you. It should *not* be taken with blood thinners.

RECOMMENDATION 2: Boost intake of folate and calcium. People who take at least 400 micrograms (mcg) of folate daily and/or 500 mg of calcium twice daily reduce their colon cancer risk by 30%. The reason for this effect is unknown, but researchers believe these supplements may slow the harmful breakdown of DNA that is associated with cancer.

MYTH: The more you exercise, the better your health. The human body isn't designed to withstand constant stress. People who exercise vigorously more than about an hour a day don't live longer or healthier lives than those who exercise at moderate levels.

RECOMMENDATION: Get one hour a day of moderate exercise —fast walking, swimming, bicycling, etc. Research shows that this level of activity can make you feel and behave younger.

Regular physical activity promotes weight loss, improves cardiovascular conditioning and bone strength and reduces the risk for diabetes.

Exercising for more than one hour doesn't provide additional health benefits but does increase the risk for muscle, bone or joint damage.

MYTH: Diarrhea should run its course. A common misconception is that it's best not to treat diarrhea in order to promote the removal of organisms/toxins that lead to this potentially dangerous condition.

Not true. Untreated diarrhea is more than just uncomfortable. It can remove quarts of water from the body and cause dangerous dehydration within 24 hours, especially in children and older adults.

RECOMMENDATION: Eat chicken soup with rice. The broth and rice provide protective sugars to cells that line the intestine. Drink two quarts of water or juice daily to prevent dehydration. Take readily absorbable, calcium-containing tablets (such as Tums) several times daily. Calcium slows muscular movements in the intestine.

■

DANGEROUS MYTHS ABOUT FEVER

Source: **Mary E. Frank, MD,** board chair and former president of the American Academy of Family Physicians. She is an associate clinical professor of ambulatory and community medicine at the University of California, San Francisco, and a family physician in private practice in Rohnert Park, CA.

If you've always believed that you can detect a fever by touching someone's forehead, then think again. The abdomen is actually more likely to feel warm when someone has a fever. However, a thermometer is the only way to accurately measure body temperature.

Here are six other common—and potentially dangerous—myths regarding fever...

MYTH 1: All adults have a normal body temperature of 98.6°F. "Normal" body temperature is conventionally said to be 98.6°F, but it actually varies. For some people, 98°F is normal, and for others, it could be 99°F. Body temperature usually rises in the course of the day—your temperature may be 98.2°F in the morning and rise to 99.4°F in late afternoon.

"Normal" temperature tends to decline with age. According to a study conducted at Yeshiva University in New York City, the average oral temperature of 150 healthy people age 65 and older was 97.5°F. Because their normal body temperature tends to be lower, some older adults may be seriously ill—even with pneumonia or a widespread infection—yet appear to have no fever at all.

MYTH 2: A fever always means that you have an infection. Not necessarily. Bacterial pneumonia or bladder infection is typically accompanied by a fever. Elevated body temperature also occurs during a number of viral illnesses, such as influenza, gastroenteritis (stomach flu)—even the common cold.

However, a fever can also signal an allergic reaction...dehydration...inflammation...a hormone disorder, such as hyperthyroidism...or an autoimmune disease, such as rheumatoid arthritis. Medications, such as antibiotics, narcotics, barbiturates and antihistamines, can trigger a fever as well. Cancer, especially leukemia or lymphoma, can cause a persistent fever of 100°F to 101°F.

MYTH 3: Fever should always be treated. Most of the time, you don't need to do anything to reduce fever. Unless it goes quite high (above 104°F in an adult), it causes no permanent damage—but you will feel uncomfortable. Some doctors suggest letting a fever run its course. That way, you won't undermine your body's natural defense process.

If you choose to let a fever run its course, drink lots of fluids to avoid becoming dehydrated by the increased metabolism that accompanies fever.

Even if you're not thirsty, keep a glass of water or juice at your bedside, and take sips often. Eat soups and suck on popsicles. Take lukewarm baths or showers.

MYTH 4: Aspirin is the best medicine for a fever. The most common *antipyretics*—fever reducers—are available over-the-counter. They include *acetaminophen* (Tylenol) and aspirin and other nonsteroidal anti-inflammatory drugs (NSAIDs), such as *ibuprofen* (Advil) and *naproxen* (Aleve).

As far as effectiveness goes, there's little difference among them—no solid evidence shows that any of these drugs works faster or better than the others in reducing fever.

IMPORTANT: Never exceed dosage recommendations without first discussing it with your physician.

Choose on the basis of your own medical profile and the medication's potential side effects...

IF YOU TAKE DAILY ASPIRIN THERAPY: Take acetaminophen. NSAIDs can undermine the benefits of aspirin therapy, according to new studies.

IF YOU HAVE HIGH BLOOD PRESSURE: Take acetaminophen. Aspirin and other NSAIDs can raise blood pressure.

IF YOU HAVE KIDNEY DISEASE: Take acetaminophen. Aspirin and other NSAIDs can damage the kidneys.

IF YOU'RE SUSCEPTIBLE TO GASTROINTESTINAL PROBLEMS: Take acetaminophen. Aspirin and other NSAIDs can irritate the digestive system and cause bleeding.

IF YOU HAVE ASTHMA: Take acetaminophen. Aspirin and other NSAIDs may trigger an attack.

IF YOU HAVE LIVER DISEASE OR DRINK MORE THAN THREE ALCOHOLIC BEVERAGES A DAY: Take aspirin or another NSAID. Acetaminophen can harm the liver in some people.

IMPORTANT: Don't give aspirin to anyone under age 15—it can cause *Reye's syndrome,* a potentially life-threatening condition that causes swelling of the brain and the degeneration of the liver.

MYTH 5: A fever means you're contagious. Not so. A person with an upper respiratory tract infection may be contagious early on, when he/she has a runny nose but no fever. On the other hand, a person can still be running a fever after several days of antibiotic treatment but no longer be contagious.

MYTH 6: All thermometers are equally accurate. Glass mercury thermometers are the most accurate but are no longer used because of potential exposure to mercury if the glass breaks. Digital oral and digital rectal thermometers are both accurate. Ear thermometers are slightly less accurate. Forehead thermometers (plastic strips that are pressed against the forehead) are not reliable for exact measurements.

IMPORTANT: Always tell your doctor which type of thermometer you used to take your temperature.

■